Keto Diet
for Beginners

The Keto Diet Recipe Book for Healthy Weight Loss
incl. Meal Prep.

[1. Edition]

Matthew Morgan

ISBN- 9781701740310

TABLE OF CONTENTS

What is the Ketogenic diet?

The ketogenic diet is essentially a feeding routine that consists of foods that have low carbohydrate content but are high in fat designed to help your body burn fat more effectively. It shares some similarities to the Atkins or low carb diet although there are subtle differences.

Feeding on a keto diet drastically reduces your carbohydrate intake and substitute it for fat. This puts your body in a state of metabolism known as Ketosis (hence the name). In this state, your body becomes conditioned to burn fat in the form of ketones for energy instead of glucose from carbohydrates.

Your liver produces ketones from breaking down fat when you eat reduces your carb intake. Ketones are broken down faster and more effectively into blood sugar & small amount of protein (which can be further broken down into glucose as well). in the absence of regular glucose, ketones become the fuel source for your body and most especially for the brain which consumes a lot of energy daily.

What this means is that one a ketogenic diet, your entire body begins to run on fat as its indirect fuel supply 24-7. This increases the rate at which your body can burn off excess fat dramatically. With time, the body not only uses up fat from food but also access fat stores in the body and burns them for energy. A keto diet is ideal for losing weight healthily without starving yourself. But it also offers several other benefits as well.

Benefits of Ketogenic Diet

Healthy weight loss: From several studies, it has been shown that a ketogenic diet is among the most effective regimens for weight loss. The diet is filling and this mean you do not starve yourself in the process. Also, with a well-planned keto diet, you do not have to bother about counting calories or tracking your food intake to lose weight at all.

Steady energy supply: your body can run effectively on ketones alone. Unlike other weight loss plans, a keto diet involves less hunger while providing a steady energy for your body and more importantly for your brain. This keeps your body strong and your brain alert.

Insulin and blood sugar control: since carbohydrate intake is replaced with fat, ketogenic diets help induce a massive reduction in insulin levels thus preventing and managing diabetes and similar conditions.

In addition to these, a ketogenic diet can also provide several health benefits for the body including reducing the risk of diseases like Alzheimer's, epilepsy, heart conditions, some types of cancer, insulin-related deficiencies among benefits.

While on a Ketogenic diet, it is recommended that you avoid high carb foods such as starches and grain, sugary foods, fruits (you can take small portions of strawberries), root veggies and tubers, beans or legumes and so on. Generally, most meals in a keto diet are based on meat, fatty fish, eggs, butter or cream, cheese, nuts & seeds, healthy oil, avocados, low-carb vegetables and so on.

Losing weight is no easy feat. To lose just 5 pounds can be quite challenging and it takes a lot of discipline and dedication. It gets even tougher when you try to do so within a short period or try to lose up to 21 pounds within 21 days. However, that's not to say it is an impossible feat. With some dietary and lifestyle changes and a lot of discipline, dedication, and patience, you can speed up your weight loss process and even do so healthily without jeopardizing your health. Here are some proven strategies that can help you lose up to 21 pounds in just 3 weeks.

1. Monitor your calorie intake: This strategy is one of most commonly used methods to lose weight fast. Using up more calories than you consume in your food is the basic principle for losing weight. To achieve this you either increase your physical activity, reduce your calorie intake or use a combination of both strategies. Of course since it is impossible to avoid calorie intake entirely, you can monitor how much calorie you take in by tracking how much calorie is in every food you put on your table contains. This, combined with activities that help you use up more calories and some other lifestyle modifications will put you on track on your incredible weight loss journey. Tracking calorie intake can be a major work. But fortunately, there are now tools to make it a lot easier. You can download an app or keep a food journal to track your calorie intake effectively.

2. More water: This is an easily overlooked strategy basically because it is so simple that most people don't know how effective it can be. However, research has shown that increasing your water intake can indeed boost your weight loss process. According to a study published in the National Center for Biotechnology Information Journal (NCBI) journal, increased water intake when paired with a low-calorie diet resulted in significantly higher weight loss in subjects over 12 weeks.

Taking more water increases the rate of metabolism and this means your body can burn calories better after each meal. Taking more water can also weight loss without even interfering with metabolism. Drinking more water during meals will help you get filled better and generally reduce food intake which is crucial for quick weight loss. It is recommended that you take as much as 34 to 68 ounces of water per day (1 to 2 liters).

3. More protein: While trying to cut down on calorie intake, it is also important that you watch what you eat and this includes upping your protein intake. It is recommended that you increase the quantity of protein-rich foods in your diet. A high-protein diet can promote weight loss while helping you to preserve your muscle mass during your weight loss journey.

Protein is also known to reduce appetite hence decreasing overall food consumption and calorie intake. Similarly, consuming a breakfast rich in protein can help reduce the production of ghrelin which is the hormone that stimulates a feeling of hunger in individuals. Therefore, you should add more protein-rich Ingredients such as meats, seafood, legumes, eggs, poultry and so on to your breakfasts and other meals of the day.

4. Cut down on carbs (especially refined carbs): Cutting down on your carbohydrate intake is vital if you must speed up your weight-loss. Refined carbs are poor in essential nutrients and have low fiber content. They have been linked several health issues including spikes in blood sugar level (due to rapid digestion), increases hunger, and most importantly weight gain and an increase in body fat.

If you intend to lose up to 21 pounds in 21 days, then you mustn't add more pounds by taking high carb meals. Food like refined grains, cereals white bread and other pre-packaged products in your diet should be removed or simply swapped for healthier alternatives. Generally, a low carb meal plan such as a Keto diet is recommended if you are serious about losing weight fast.

5. Start resistance training: Everyone knows working out is a basic requirement for weight loss. However, for even quicker weight-loss, there are specific exercise regimes that are recommended for you. Resistance training is a form of exercise routine that involves working against a resistive force. These types of exercise not only increase endurance and muscle strength but are also effective for burning up excess fat as well. They can also speed up the rate of metabolism thereby helping you to burn more calories. You can hit the gym or simply try resistance routines like planks, squats, and lunges right at home.

6. More fiber: As part of watching what you eat, adding more fiber to your meals will help in your quest to lose weight fast. Fibers slow down the rate of digestion and keep your stomach full for longer. This ability to keep you satiated will reduce food intake which will score you big points in terms of weight control ad reduced calorie intake. You should add more fruits, whole grains, nuts, seeds, and veggies to your daily diet as an integral part of your fat weight-loss regimen.

7. Sleep: While this might sound counter-intuitive, several weight-loss studies suggest that a healthy sleep schedule is important to your quest to lose weight just as much as diet and exercise is. Not getting enough sleep can cause you to pack on more pounds. Sleep deprivation has also been linked to elevated hunger due to the increased production of hunger hormones. This boosts appetite and can lead to weight gain in the long run. While you may not need more sleep, establishing a healthy and consistent sleep cycle will keep you healthy and increase weight loss.

8. Mindfulness: This strategy isn't so much of a scientific one, but it is quite effective too. Mindfulness involves practicing being aware of your feelings and thoughts while focusing on your present moments. Experts recommend slow eating while practicing mindfulness as one of the tricks to decrease food intake. Most people chew through their meals fast without paying attention to how and what they eat. Staying focused while you eat, taking time to chew your food and practicing mindfulness is recommended for healthy feeding and resultant weight loss. You will also enjoy your food better.

9. Monitor your progress: as earlier mentioned, losing weight is no easy feat and even harder if you want to do so within a limited time. You will have to keep a strict eye on your journey to avoid any slip-ups. People who weigh themselves daily are more likely to stay conscious of their weight-loss plan compared to those who do so less frequently. You can also keep a food journal or use apps to track your progress. You can practice staying accountable by joining a weight-loss community or simply taking up the challenge with a friend or simply share your 21-days journey to losing 21 pounds with friends online. This will provide the motivation you need to keep up.

Bottom line

Losing 21 pounds in 3 weeks may seem like an impossible challenge. But it is achievable when you know the right strategies to use. Of course, one of the biggest challenges is losing weight within such a short period without compromising your health. By following the guide above, doing both should be a lot easier.

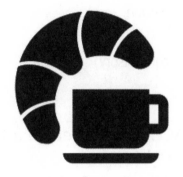

Time: 40 minutes | Amount: 12 yields

Calories: 217 kcal | Carbs: 6g | Protein:7g | Fat:19g

Ingredients

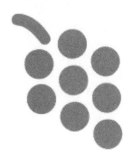

- Almond flour (2 1/2 c)
- Keto friendly sugar (e.g. Swerve) (2 1/2 c)
- Kosher salt ((1/2 tsp)
- Baking soda (1/2 tsp)
- Baking powder (1.5 teaspoon)
- Melted butter (1/3c)
- Eggs (3 large)
- Unsweetened almond milk (1/3 c)
- Vanilla extract (pure) 1 teaspoon
- fresh blueberries (2/3c)
- Zest from 1/2 lemon (not compulsory)

How to prepare

1.	Heat oven to 350º/180oC. Prepare a 12-cup muffin pan by lining with cupcake liners
2.	Mix the almond flour, baking powder, sugar, salt and baking soda. Also whisk melted butter, almond milk, eggs and vanilla into the mixture until well combined
3.	Gently fold-in blueberries till it is distributed evenly in the mixture. (also add lemon zest if desired). Scoop equal amount of batter into each cupcake liner. Bake for 23 minutes till it is slightly golden and it passes the toothpick test.
4.	Allow to cool slightly before you serve

Ingredients

- Almond milk (3/4c)
- Ice (1/2c)
- Almond butter (2 tablespoons)
- Unsweetened cocoa powder (2 tablespoons)
- Swerve or any other keto friendly sugar (2-3 tablespoons)
- Chia seeds (1 tablespoon and more for serving)
- Hemp seeds (2 tablespoons and more for serving)
- Vanilla extract-pure (1/2 tablespoon)
- Kosher salt (a pinch)

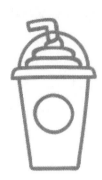

How to prepare

1.	In a blender, mix all your Ingredients until smooth.
2.	Pour mixture into a glass then add chia and hemp seeds as garnish.

Time: 20 Minutes | Amount: 3 yields

Calories: 132 kcal | Carbs: 2g | Protein: 10g | Fat: 9g

Ingredients

♦ Bell pepper (1, sliced into rings of 1/4")
♦ 6 eggs
♦ Black peppers (freshly ground)
♦ Kosher salt
♦ Chopped parsley (2 tablespoons)
♦ Chopped chives (2 tablespoons)

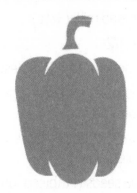

How to prepare

1.	Over medium heat, place a skillet then grease lightly with some cooking spray
2.	Place the bell pepper rings in skillet. Saute for 2 to 3 minutes
3.	Flip rings and crack an egg in the middle. Add salt & pepper then cook until egg is well cooked (for 2-4 minutes)
4.	Repeat for other eggs. To be served garnished with chives and parsley.

Time: 35 Minutes | Amount: 3 cups
Calories:244kcal | Carbs: 9g | Protein: 4g | Fat: 22g

Ingredients

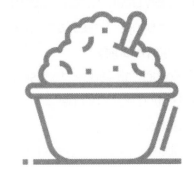

- Chopped almonds (1c)
- Chopped walnuts (1c)
- Coconut flakes-unsweetened (1c)
- Sesame seeds (1/4c)
- Flax seeds (2 tablespoon)
- Chia seeds (1/2tsp)
- Ground clove (1/2tsp)
- Cinnamon-ground (1 1/2 tsp)
- Kosher salt (1/2 tsp)
- Melted coconut oil (1/4 c)
- Vanilla extract (1 tsp, pure)
- Egg white (from one egg)

How to prepare

1.	Heat the oven to about 350°F/180oC . prepare baking sheet by spraying with cooking spray.
2.	Mix almonds, coconut flakes, walnuts, flax seeds, sesame & chia seeds in a bowl.
3.	Stir in the cinnamon, cloves, vanilla extract & salt
4.	Beat egg white until it become foamy then stir into the granola. Add some coconut oil then stir till it is well-coated
5.	Pour onto the baking sheet, spreading evenly
6.	Bake this for 20 -24 minutes or until it starts to turn golden. You can stir gently halfway through cooking.
7.	Leave to Cool for a short while, then serve.

Time: 15 minutes | Amount: 3 servings

Calories: 603 kcal | Carbs:7g | Protein: 22g | Fat: 54g

Ingredients

- Heavy cream (2 tablespoon)
- Red pepper flakes (a pinch)
- Eggs (6 large)
- Kosher salt (added to taste)
- Ground black pepper
- Butter (1 tbsp)
- Sliced cheddar (2 slices)
- Frozen patties (6)
- Sliced Avocado

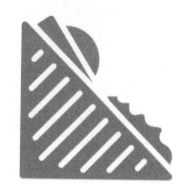

How to prepare

1.	Beat the eggs, red pepper flakes & heavy cream in a bowl.
2.	Add salt & pepper according to your preference.
3.	Melt butter in a skillet over medium heat
4.	Pour some of the egg mixture (about 1/3) into skillet
5.	In the middle of this, place a slice of cheese and leave for 1 minute.
6.	Fold-in the sides of the egg to cover the cheese in the middle
7.	Remove from pan. Repeat the same process for the remaining egg mixture
8.	To be serve with two sausage patties and Avocado.

Time: 7 minutes | Amount: 6 burritos
Calories: 331 kcal | Carbs :1g | Proteins:11g | Fat: 30g

Ingredients

- Butter (6 tbsp)
- Eggs (12 medium)
- Cream (12 tablespoons)
- Salt and pepper (added to taste)
- Herbs and spices of choice

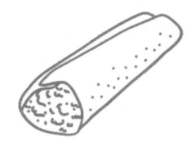

How to prepare

1.	Whisk eggs, cream and any herbs and spices in a small bowl
2.	Melt butter in frying pan. Pour in the egg mixture
3.	Swirl frying pan until the content is evenly spread and as thin as possible
4.	Cover pan with a lid then cook for about 2 minutes
5.	Gently life burrito from frying pan with a spatula
6.	Can be served rolled up with any fillings of your choice

Time: 25 Minutes | Amount: 4 wraps

Calories: 637kcal | Carbs:14g | Protein:31g | Fat: 51g

Ingredients

- Chicken sausages (4)
- Eggs (8 to 9 large)
- Hass Avocado (2, ripe and soft)
- Jalapeno cream cheese-softened (8 tablespoons)
- Butter (4 teaspoon)
- Pepper and salt

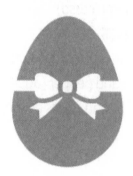

How to prepare

1.	Place chicken sausages in medium skillet over medium to high heat. Sear for a while to warm through. Transfer sausages to a plate. Cover with a foil. Set aside to cool. Wipe skillet with paper tower.
2.	Crack eggs into a bowl, add 1/2 teaspoon salt and 1/4 teaspoon black pepper. Whisk egg thoroughly until it forms a foam
3.	Place 1 tsp butter into skillet. Leave to melt then add 1/2 cup eggs. Swirl egg in the pan to form a 11 to 12 inch circle. Cook for 1 to 2 minutes. Then flip over using a large spatula. Cook this for 30 to 60 more seconds
4.	Slide egg crepe onto cutting board. Do this for remaining egg mixture as well. You should have 4 egg wraps in total.
5.	On each wrap, scoop half of an avocado and spread into a thin layer. Spread 2 tbsp of jalapeno cream cheese over avocado.
6.	On each egg wrap, place one chicken sausage then fold the wrap over with the sides folding inward like a burrito. Tuck the sides neatly as you roll. Repeat for all four rolls
7.	To be served warm

Time:25 minutes | Amount: 2 servings

Calories: 663 kcal | Carbs:4g | Proteins:28g | Fats: 59g

Ingredients

- Diced halloumi cheese (3 oz/74g)
- Diced Scallions (2)
- Olive oil (2 tbsp)
- Diced bacon (4 oz/102g)
- Fresh chopped parsley (4 tablespoon)
- 4 eggs
- Pitted olives (1/2 cup)
- Salt and pepper

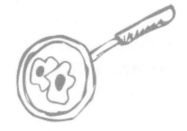

How to prepare

1.	Heat oil over high heat in a medium frying pan. Fry halloumi, bacon and scallions in the oil till they are nicely browned
2.	Whisk eggs and parsley in a small bowl. Add salt and pepper to season
3.	Pour your egg mixture into the frying pan over the bacon & cheese mixture.
4.	Lower heat & add olives. Stir for some minutes until it is done to your preference.

KETO SCRAMBLED EGGS WITH HALLOUMI CHEESE

Time: 40 minutes | Amount:12 Yields

Calories:137 kcal | Carbs: 1g | Protein: 6g | fat: 64g

Ingredients

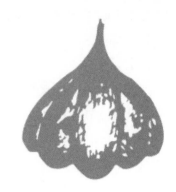

- Ground pork (2 lbs/0.9 kg)
- Freshly chopped thyme (1 tablespoon)
- Garlic (2cloves)-Minced
- Paprika (1/2 teaspoon)
- Ground cumin (2 1/2 tsp)
- Kosher salt (1 tsp)
- 12 eggs
- Fresh spinach (2 1/2 cup)
- Fresh ground pepper
- shredded white cheddar (1 cup)
- Chives (freshly chopped) 1 tablespoon

How to prepare

1.	Preheat the oven to about 400oF/202oC
2.	Mix ground pork, thyme, paprika, cumin, garlic & salt in a bowl. add black pepper to season.
3.	Add a small handful of pork mixture to muffin tin then create a cup by pressing up the sides.
4.	Add spinach and cheese divided evenly between the cups. On top of each cup, crack an egg then add a pinch of salt & pepper.
5.	Bake for 25 minutes till eggs are set and sausage is well cooked. Garnish with chives then serve

Time: 25 minutes | Amount: 1 servings

Calories: 360kcal | Carbs:4g | Protein: 20g | Fat:29g

Ingredients

- Aged heddar (Tilamook) (3 oz/ 78g)
- 1 large egg (pastured)
- Sugar free bacon (pastured)- 2 slices
- Cilantro (2 sprigs)
- Arugula (a handful)
- Ghee (1 teaspoon)
- Salt, pepper and turmeric (a pinch)

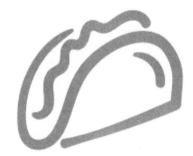

How to prepare

1.	Cook bacon by frying or baking in oven until it is crispy. Set aside
2.	Shred cheese with a cheese grater.
3.	Over medium heat, skillet then add ghee. Sprinkle cheese into skill over the ghee forming a circle
4.	Once cheese melts & becomes bubbly, crack egg into the skillet in the center of the circle. Sprinkle some salt, pepper & turmeric on the yolk
5.	Cook for 2 minutes till egg starts turning opaque and cheese starts to brown
6.	Cover and cook for about 2 more minutes.
7.	Remove from the heat. The eggs should be fully cooked and cheese should be crispy.
8.	Carefully slid onto a dish or cutting board. Hold sides of the taco sheet up with two bowls or cups. This way the sides of the sheet remains up as its shell cools.
9.	Add bacon, cilantro and arugula.

Time: 15 minutes | Amount: 10 yields
Calories: 360kcal | Carbs:4g | Protein: 20g | Fat:29g

Ingredients

- Almond flour (1/2 cup)
- Softened cream cheese (4 oz/102g)
- 4 large eggs
- lemon zest (1 teaspoon)
- Butter (for frying & serving)

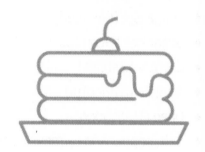

How to prepare

1.	Whisk almond flour, eggs, cream cheese & lemon zest in a bowl. Mix till smooth
2.	In a skillet, melt 1 tablespoon of butter over medium heat. Pour in 3 tablespoons of batter and cook for about 2 minutes or till it turns golden.
3.	Flip then for 2 additional minutes.
4.	Transfer to serving plate and leave aside while you cook the remaining portion of the batter.
5.	Serve with butter as topping.

Time: 40 minutes | Amount: 8 servings
Calories: 35kcal | Carbs:-0.4g | Protein: 2.2g | Fat: 2.8g

Ingredients

♦ 3 large eggs

♦ Tarter cream (1/2 teaspoon)

♦ Kosher salt (a pinch)

♦ Softened cream cheese (2 oz.)

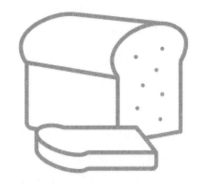

How to prepare

1.	Heat oven to about 300oF/150oC. Prepare a large baking sheet by lining with parchment paper
2.	Separate yolks from & put in two different glass bowls.
3.	To the egg white add some cream of tarter & salt. Beat this until stiff peaks for 3 minutes.
4.	To egg yolk, add cream cheese them mix until well combined using a hand mixer.
5.	Gently fold egg yolk mixture into egg white
6.	Divide the mixture formed into 8 mounds and place on a baking sheet. Leave a spacing of about 4" in between them.
7.	Bake in oven for about 30 minutes or till color turns golden
8.	Sprinkle each piece some cheese on each bread & bake for about 2 minutes till cheese begins to melt. Leave for a while to cool before serving

Time: 20 minutes | Amount: 4 servings

Calories: 126kcal | Carbs:5g | Protein: 3g | Fat:10g

Ingredients

- Turnip (1 large) peeled then diced
- Onion-diced (1/4)
- Brussel sprouts (halved)-1 cup
- Bacon (3 slices)
- Olive oil (1 tbsp)
- Garlic powder (1/2 teaspoon)
- Paprika (1/2 teaspoon)
- Black pepper (1/2 teaspoon)
- Parsley (1 tbsp)-for garnish
- Diced red bell pepper (1/4 cup)
- Salt (1/2 teaspoon)

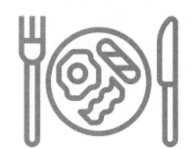

How to prepare

1.	To a large skillet over medium to high heat skillet, add oil.
2.	Add turnips and other spices
3.	Cook for 5 to 7 minutes. Stir continuously as you cook
4.	Add onion and brussel sprouts. Cook for about 3 minutes till softened
5.	Chop bacon into small pieces. Add to skillet along with the red bell pepper
6.	Cook for 5 to 7 more minutes until bacon is well cooked
7.	Serve garnished with parsley

Time:1 hour | Amount: 4 yields

Calories: 223kcal | Carbs:4g | Protein: 21g | Fat:27g

Ingredients

- ◆ Bell peppers (2 halved and seeded)
- ◆ 8 eggs (lightly beaten)
- ◆ Milk (1/4 cup)
- ◆ Cooked and crumbled bacon (4 slices)
- ◆ Shredded cheddar (1 cup)
- ◆ Chives (finely chopped) (2 tablespoon + more for garnish)
- ◆ Black pepper
- ◆ Kosher salt

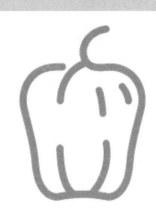

How to prepare

1.	Preheat the oven to 400oF/ 202oC
2.	Place the halved bell peppers in the baking dish with cut side up
3.	Add water to the dish then place in the oven for about 5 minutes
4.	Beat egg & milk in a bowl. Add bacon, chives and cheese. Season with pepper & salt.
5.	When peppers are done, divide the egg mixture into the peppers. Return peppers into oven then bake for about 35 minutes more until the eggs are set. Serve with more chives.

Time: 45 minutes | Amount: 4 servings

Calories: 661 kcal | Carbs:4g | Protein: 27g | Fat:59g

Ingredients

- Bacon or chorizo (diced) 5 oz/130g
- Butter (2 tablespoon)
- Fresh spinach (8oz/204g)
- 8 eggs
- Heavy cream (1 cup)
- Shredded cheese (5 oz/130g)
- Salt & pepper

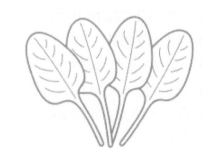

How to prepare

1.	Heat your oven to 350ºF or 175ºC.
2.	Grease the baking dish
3.	Fry bacon in better over medium heat.
4.	Add spinach then stir until it is wilted
5.	Remove pan from heat then set aside
6.	Whisk eggs with cream and pour into the ramekins or baking dish
7.	Add bacon, cheese and prepared spinach as topping. Place baking dish into the oven then bake for 30 minutes till the top turns a golden color.

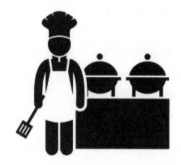

Time: 35 minutes | Amount: 6 servings

Calories: 359kcal | Carbs: 6.7g | Protein:34.4g | Fat:23g

Ingredients

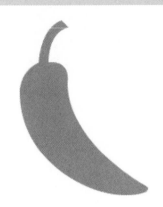

- Avocado oil (1/2 tablespoon)
- 2 ribs celery (chopped)
- Ground beef-85/15 (2 lbs/0.9kg)
- Chipotle chilli powder (1 teaspoon)
- Cumin (1 tablespoon)
- Garlic powder (2 teaspoon)
- Salt (1 teaspoon)
- Black pepper (1 teaspoon)
- Tomato sauce (1, 15oz/425g can)-no salt added
- Beef bone broth (16 oz container/480g)
- Optional garnishes: cheddar cheese, sour cream, sliced jalapeno, green onion, cilantro

How to prepare

1.	Heat avocado oil over medium heat in a large pot. Add the chopped celery & cook for 3-4 minutes until softened. Set aside in a small bowl
2.	Add beef, brown beef and spices in the same pot and cook till it is well cooked throughout
3.	Turn down the heat then add the tomato sauce and beef bone broth to cooked beef. Leave to simmer for about 10 additional minutes. Stir occasionally.
4.	Return celery to the pot. Stir till it is thoroughly mixed-in.
5.	Garnish and serve

Time: 50 Minutes | Amount: 4 servings

Calories: 568 kcal | Carbs: 6g | Protein: 39g | Fat: 40.2g

Ingredients

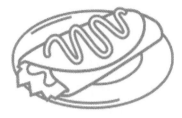

- Coconut oil (2 tablespoons)
- Chicken thighs (Boneless &skinless)
- Enchilada sauce (3/4 cup)
- Water (1/4 cup)
- Onion (1/4 cup)
- Green chilies (1 can 4 oz/113g)
- For toppings(customize according to choice)
- Avocado (1, diced)
- Shredded cheese (1c)
- Picked jalapenos (1/4c)
- Roma tomato (1, chopped)
- Sour cream (1/2 c)

How to prepare

1.	Sear the chicken thighs in a pot or dutch over over medium to high heat until it is lightly browned.
2.	Pour in the enchilada sauce, add water then onion & green chilies. Turn the heat down, cover then leave to simmer for 17 to 25 minutes until chicken becomes tender and well cooked through
3.	Remove chicken carefully then chop or shred. Return chopped chicken to the pot then simmer again for 10 more minutes
4.	Served with desired toppings. Can be served alone or with cauliflower rice

Time: 20 Minutes | Amount:4 servings
Calories: 202 kcal | Carbs:7g | Protein: 3g | Fat: 18g

Ingredients

- Cucumber (2 large, about 10 oz/280g each)
- For tahini sauce
- Tahini (1/4 cup)
- Olive oil, extra-virgin (3 tablespoons)
- Water (3 tbps)
- Garlic cloves (2)
- Cumin (1/4 tsp)
- Lemon juice (1 1/2 tablespoon)
- Sea salt & black pepper
- Smoked paprika (1/8 tsp)

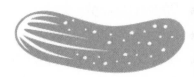

How to prepare

1.	Put all Ingredients for the tahini sauce in blender and puree till it attains a smooth consistency. If too thick, you can add water 1 tbsp at a time to it until it is as thin as desired.
2.	Spiralize cucumbers with a spiralizer. Add salt as desired then set over sink to drain
3.	Pat cucumber noddles. Serve into plates and drizzle with the prepared tahini sauce.

Time: 15 Minutes | Amount: 6 servings

Calories: 69kcal | Carbs: 2.7g | Protein:1.1g | Fat: 9g

Ingredients

- Raw boneless white f ish (1 lb/0.45kg)
- Salt (a pinch)
- Chilli flakes (a pinch)
- Cilantro stems and leaves (1/4 cup)
- Garlic cloves (not compulsory)
- Coconut oil or ghee (1 or 2 tablespoons)
- Avocado oil (for greasing hands)
- For the sauce:
- 2 ripe avocados
- Juice(from 1 lemon)
- Salt
- Water (2 tablespoons)

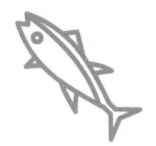

How to prepare

1.	Add fish, herbs, salt and chilli into food processor then blitz until it is well mixed
2.	To a frying pan over medium to high heat add some coconut oil. Swirl pan around till all sides are coated.
3.	Oil your hands. Roll fish mixture into 6 patties
4.	Add patties to the heated frying pan. Cook both sides till they turn a light golden brown color.
5.	Add Ingredients for the dipping sauce into the food processor or blender then blitz until it is smooth & creamy.
6.	Serve fish cakes warm with the sauce.

Time: 1 hr 15 min | Amount: 8 servings

Calories: 160 kcal | Carbs:4g | Protein: 16g | Fat: 13g

Ingredients

- Olive oil (about 350ml)
- White onion (4oz/110g)
- Radishes (peeled & thinly sliced, crosswise) 700g/24oz
- Kosher salt (added to taste)
- 8 eggs
- Black pepper (freshly ground)
- Fresh parsley (as garnish)

How to prepare

1.	Heat up some of the olive oil over medium heat in a frying pan.
2.	Once it begins to simmer, turn the heat down. Add radish & onion slices. Season with salt and layer them on your pan. Be sure to stir occasionally as you cook for 37 to 45 minutes until it is tender and silky smooth.
3.	Whisk egg lightly with a generous amount of salt while radishes are cooking.
4.	Once cooked, drain radishes and onions, cool for some minutes. Pour in the eggs.
5.	Grease a non-stick pan lightly with the reserved oil. Radish and egg mixture & cook for 3 minutes until the sides start to set.
6.	Turn the heat off & leave the pan covered for about 5 minutes.
7.	After five minutes, remove pan from the heat. Place a large plat to cover the skillet then set your hands on top and invert the tortilla onto it (do this over the sink)
8.	Add olive oil to pan (1 or 3 tablespoons). Slowly slide tortilla back onto the skillet from the plate. Cook for about 4 more minutes until the second side becomes lightly browned.
9.	Invert tortilla back onto a clean plate. Leave to cool for 10 minutes then serve.

Time: 45 minutes | Amount: 6 servings

Calories: 409 kcal | Carbs :8g | Proteins:16g | Fat: 34g

Ingredients

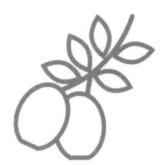

- Coconut oil (3 tablespoons)
- 6 slices of bacon (about 168g/6oz)
- Bell peppers (2 medium, 8.5oz/240g)-diced
- Spinach (4 cups) chopped
- Tomatoes (2 small) diced
- 12 eggs (whisked)
- Basil leaves (1/4 cup)
- 15 olives (diced)
- 3 cloves of Minced & finely diced garlic
- Pepper and salt (added to taste)
- Coconut cream (3/4 cup)

How to prepare

1.	Preheat oven to 175oC or 350oF
2.	Melt coconut oil over medium/high heat in a skillet Saute bacon for 4 minutes. Remove sauteed bacon using a slotted spoon then set aside.
3.	Add onion & bell pepper along with the the bacon fat into same skillet and saute for about 5 minutes
4.	Add spinach, and saute for 1 or 2 minutes till it is wilted. Remove from heat then set aside and leave to cool.
5.	Mix tomato, eggs, basil, olives, coconut cream, bacon, garlic and spinach mixture in a bowl. Add salt and pepper to season. Pour mixture into a square baking dish (about 9" by 9" or 23cm by 23cm).
6.	Bake for about 30 minutes. Remove and serve

Time: 10 Minutes | Amount: 2 wraps

Calories: 161 kcal | Carbs: 8g | Protein: 11g | Fat: 10g

Ingredients

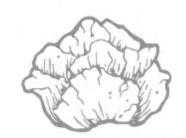

- ◆ Cooked & chopped center cut bacon (4 slices)
- ◆ Tomato, diced (1 medium)
- ◆ Light mayonnaise (1 tablespoon)
- ◆ Iceberg lettuce leaves (3 large)
- ◆ Fresh black pepper
- ◆ Avocado (1 oz/28g)-optional

How to prepare

1.	Remove 2 large outer leaves of a lettuce head as carefully as possible and set aside. Remove a third leave and shred/
2.	Dice tomato and leave aside in a bowl
3.	Mix diced tomato with mayonnaise with black pepper
4.	Place the lettuce cups on the serving plate. Top this with the shredded lettuce then add tomato mixture and bacon then roll it like a wrap.

Time:20 minutes | Amount: 16 tortillas
Calories: 50 kcal | Carbs:6g | Proteins: 8.5g | Fats: 1.5g

Ingredients

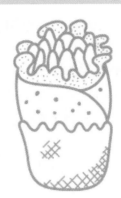

- Egg whites (from 8 large eggs)
- Coconut flour (1/3c)
- Water (10 tablespoon)
- Baking powder and onion powder (1/4 tsp each)
- Garlic powder and Chilli powder (1/4 tsp each)
- Chilli powder (1/4 tsp)
- Himalayan salt (1/4 tsp)

How to prepare

1.	Combine egg whites, baking powder, coconut flour & water in a bowl. Mix well till it forms a uniform watery mixture. You may add seasoning to this if you desire.
2.	Heat skillet on low heat, wait till pan is slightly hot then spray with the cooking spray.
3.	Drop some of this mixture into skillet (Use a 1/4 cup measuring cup)
4.	Swivel skillet around as quickly as possible to spread this batter as thin as you can. Add more to the areas not well covered.
5.	Cook for some minutes till it begins to rise or when the underside is browned. Flip then cook this side for 1additional minute
6.	Repeat this same process until all the batter has been well cooked. You should get 16 taco-sized tortillas from this.

Time: 5 minutes | Amount: 2 servings

Calories:116kcal | Carbs: 2g | Protein: 1g | Fat: 12g

Ingredients

- 1 Cucumber (about 220g/7oz.) sliced then quartered
- Mayo (2 tbsp)
- Lemon juice (2 tbsp)
- Fresh ground black pepper & salt

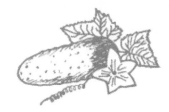

How to prepare

1.	Mix cucumber slices, lemon juice & mayo in a small bowl
2.	Add salt & pepper as desired

Time:50 minutes | Amount: 10 servings
Calories: 261kcal | Carbs:6g | Protein: 17g | Fat:18g

Ingredients

- 90% lean ground beef (2 lbs/0.9kg)
- Onion (1/4 large) diced
- Garlic (1 clove) mined
- Ground cumin (1 teaspoon)
- 1 head cabbage (large, chopped)
- Bullion (4 cubes)
- Rotel diced tomatoes and green chilies (1 can 280g/10 oz)
- Salt and pepper (added to taste)
- Water (4 cups)

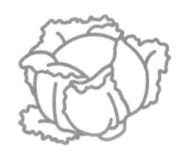

How to prepare

1.	Brown ground beef over medium to high heat.
2.	Add onion & cook for a while till it is softened and translucent
3.	Transfer onion and beef mixture to stock pot
4.	Add in garlic, cumin, bullion cubes, diced tomatoes and chillies, water and the bouillon cubes into the stock pot
5.	Mix thoroughly and bring as you boil over high heat
6.	Reduce heat & leave to simmer over low heat for about 30 to 45 minutes.

Calories:302 kcal | Carbs: 27g | Protein: 5g | Fat: 7g

Ingredients

- Cauliflower, cut into florets (2 heads, 10 cups of florets)
- Olive oil (2 tablespoons)
- Sea salt (1/2 teaspoon)
- Avocado mayonnaise (1.5 cups)
- Diced dill pickles (1 cup)
- Diced celery (1/2 cup)
- Hard boiled eggs (6 large)
- 1 tbsp Apple cider vinegar
- Black pepper
- Paprika (for topping)

How to prepare

1.	Preheat oven to 180oC/375oF. Prepare two baking sheets by lining them with parchment paper
2.	Dice cauliflower into cubes about an inch each and toss with olive oil, pepper and salt
3.	Spread this onto baking sheets (spread in a single layer). Bake in preheated oven for about 30 minutes. Flip as soon as the tips turn golden. Leave to cool
4.	Meanwhile, hard boil the eggs and dice 4 of them and slice the remaining 2
5.	In a bowl, mix all remaining Ingredients then add it to the cauliflower and diced eggs. Toss until well coated. You should taste it to see if more pepper & salt is needed . Layer into a serving dish then lay the sliced eggs on top.
6.	Serve sprinkled with paprika and chilli

Time: 7 hours 30 minutes (30 minutes of active time) | Amount: 2-3 servings

Calories:656kcal | Carbs:1.4g | Protein:50.2g | Fat:48.5g

Ingredients

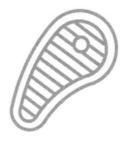

- Pastured beef (beef shank or short ribs) (3.5 lbs/ 1.6kg)
- Turmeric (2 teaspoons)
- Salt (1 teaspoon)
- Pepper (1/2 teaspoon)
- Cumin (2 teaspoons)
- Coriander (2 teaspoons)
- Water (1/2 cup)
- Coarsely chopped Cilantro stems (1 cup)
- Crushed garlic (4 cloves)- optional
- Chipotle powder (1 teaspoon)-optional
- Paprika (2 teaspoons)- optional

How to prepare

1.	Mix all your dry ingredient in a small bowl. Add the short rib to this mixture and coat then place in a slow cooker
2.	Sprinkle cilantro stems and garlic over the ribs if you are using it. Add water (do this carefully so that spices are not rinsed off)
3.	Cook in slow cooker for about 6 to 7 hour. You should check after 6 hours to see if meat is tender enough
4.	Drain cooking liquid into a saucepan. Heat on medium heat for 15 additional minutes. Return this liquid to the pot. Pull meat apart with forks and shred the beef.
5.	Can be served hot with guacamole, roasted pumpkin, fresh cilantro or green beans.

Time: 10minutes | Amount: 2 servings

Calories: 575kcal | Carbs:11g | Protein: 45g g | Fat:29g

Ingredients

- ◆ For lemon dressing
- ◆ Olive oil (1/4 cup)
- ◆ Lemon juice (2 tablespoons)
- ◆ Dijon mustard (1 teaspoon)
- ◆ Black pepper
- ◆ White wine vinegar (1 teaspoon)
- ◆ For salad
- ◆ Arugula (3 oz/ 85g)
- ◆ Cooked salmon fillets (8 oz/226g)
- ◆ 1 avocado

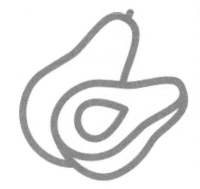

How to prepare

1.	Mix all Ingredients for the dressing together in a bowl or jug vigorously until it becomes emulsified.
2.	To prepare salad, add arugula leaves, diced avocado and flaked salmon into a serving bowl.
3.	Toss gently then drizzle with some of the lemon dressing

Time:2 hour (50 active minutes) | Amount: 12 slices
Calories: 77kcal | Carbs:1g | Protein: 7g | Fat:5g

Ingredients

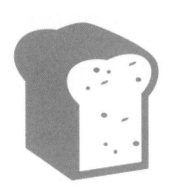

- Collagen protein (grass-fed, unflavored)
- Almond flour (6 tablespoons)
- Pastured eggs (5, separated)
- Coconut oil (1 tablespoon) unflavored
- Baking powder (1 teaspoon) aluminum free
- Xanthan gum (1 teaspoon)
- Himalayan pink salt (a pinch)
- Stevia (a pinch)-optional

How to prepare

1.	Preheat your oven to 325oF/160oC
2.	Oil the base of a ceramic load dish (standard size) with some coconut oil (ghee or butter can be used as well) or simply cover the bottom of the dish with parchment paper
3.	Beat egg whites until it foams then lay aside.
4.	Mix all dry Ingredients in a bowl. A pinch of stevia can be added to offset the egg flavor if you don't like it
5.	Mix egg yolks & coconut oil in a different bowl
6.	Mix all the dry and wet Ingredients until it is well combined. Your batter should be a little gooey but thick.
7.	Pour batter into lined dish and place inside the oven
8.	Bake for 40 minutes then remove from oven and set aside to cool for 1 to 2 hours.
9.	Release from the dish then cut bread into 12 even slices.

Time: 2hrs 30 min | Amount: 6 servings

Calories: 288 kcal | Carbs:8g | Protein: 20g | Fat:20g

Ingredients

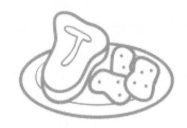

- Beef chuck roast (trimmed & cubed) 1.25 lbs/0.6kg
- Whole mushrooms (8 oz/226g) quartered
- Celery root-6oz/180g (peeled & cubed into smaller pieces about 3/4 inches each)
- Pearl onions (trimmed & peeled (4 oz/226g)
- Carrots (3 oz/80g)
- Tomato paste (2 tablespoon)
- Ribs celery (2 or 3) sliced
- Olive oil, bacon grease or avocado oil (2 tablespoon)
- Beef broth (5 cups)
- Bay leaf (1, large)
- Thyme (1/2 teaspoon)
- Pepper and salt (added to taste)
- Other seasoning of choice

How to prepare

1.	Remove chuck roast from the refrigerator and bring to room temperature. Trim off excess fat by pot roasting and cut into cubes (about 1 inch per cube). mix 2 teaspoons of oil into beef
2.	Wash and cut mushrooms and other vegetables including the garlic to required size. Set mushroom aside in a bowl and the other veggies in a different bowl
3.	Add oil to a dutch oven or heavy bottom pot on a stove over medium heat. Swirl the oil around to completely coat the pot bottom. Add in the mushroom and stir lightly to coat then leave for about 2 minutes without stirring. After two minutes, stir, then leave for 2 more minutes. Remove mushrooms from pot and transfer to the bowl with other vegetables.
4.	Brown beef in the pot. Do this in batches. You can add more oil if desired
5.	Placed all the browned beef in the pot then add seasoning and tomato paste to coat. Leave for about a minute more to cook then add 1 cup of the broth. Cover for about 1.5 hours with the heat turned down to low. You can add the rest up the broth as the stew simmer.
6.	Once tender, add the vegetables and turn up heat to simmer for 40 more minutes then add salt & pepper.

LOW CARB BEEF STEW

43

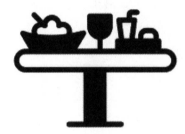

Ingredients

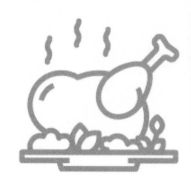

- 4 large chicken breasts (large)
- Butter (1 tablespoon_
- Chicken broth (2 cups)
- Canned diced tomatoes (10 oz/280g)- undrained
- 1/2 onion (chopped)
- Tomato paste (2 oz/56g)
- Chilli powder (1 tablespoon)
- Cumin (1 tablespoon)
- Jalapeno pepper (1, chopped) optional
- Garlic powder (1/2 tablespoon)
- Cream cheese (4 oz/102g)
- Pepper & salt (to taste)

How to prepare

1.	Boil or broth chicken breast for 10 on a stove-top. Cook till it is no longer pink then remove from fluid. Shred using two forks (alternatively, you can use a pressure cooker to cook for 5 minutes or use a slow cooker about for 4-6 hrs)
2.	Melt butter inside a stockpot over medium to high heat. Cook along with onions until it turns translucent.
3.	To this, add the shredded chicken along with the broth, diced tomatoes, chilli powder, tomato paste, garlic powder, cumin and jalapeno. Gently mix over the burner.
4.	Bring this to boil then cover and turn down the heat for about10 minutes.
5.	Cut cream cheese into small chunks (about 1 inch)
6.	Remove lid then mix-in the cream cheese.
7.	Increase heat to medium to high and stir continuously to blend in the cream cheese.
8.	Remove pot from heat then add salt and pepper to season
9.	Serve with any desired toppings.

SHREDDED CHICKEN CHILI

Time: 20 Minutes | Amount: 6 yields

Calories 410 kcal | Carbs: 4g | Protein: 26g | Fat: 20g

Ingredients

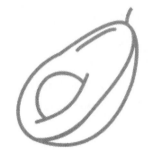

- Ground beef (0.45kg/1 lb)
- Chilli powder (1 tbsp)
- Salt (1/2 tsp)
- Cumin (3/4 tsp)
- Garlic powder (1/4 teaspoon)
- Tomato sauce (4 oz/02g)
- Dried oregano (1/2tsp)
- Onion powder (1/2 tsp)
- Avocados (3, halved)
- Cheddar cheese (1 cup) shredded
- Cherry tomatoes (sliced, 1/4 cup)
- Lettuce (shredded) 1/4 cup
- Cilantro & sour cream(as toppings)

How to prepare

1.	Cook the ground beef over medium heat in a saucepan till lightly browned
2.	Drain grease and add seasonings and tomato sauce. Stir gently to combine & cook for 4 minutes
3.	Pit halved avocados. In the crater left after pitting, Load taco meat and top with cheese, lettuce, tomatoes, sour cream and cilantro.
4.	You can make a larger area in the avocado by spooning out more it and setting this aside to make guacamole.

Time: 20 Minutes | Amount: 4 servings

Calories: 410 kcal | Carbs: 11g | Protein: 45g | Fat: 18g

Ingredients

- Coconut butter (1/2 teaspoon)
- Diced onion (1, medium)
- Chicken fillets (about 500g/20oz)
- Garlic (1, minced)
- Zucchinis (2, medium)
- Crushed tomatoes (16oz/400g)
- Cherry tomatoes (chopped in half) 7 to 10
- Raw cashews (4oz/100g)
- Seasonings (turmeric, salt, pepper, dry oregano, basil, and paprika)

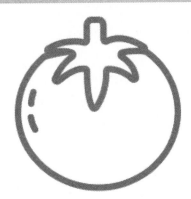

How to prepare

1.	Heat a large skillet an over medium to high heat. Add coconut butter & diced onions & cook for 1 minute or less. Ensure that you don't burn onions
2.	Dice chicken into smaller pieces and add into a pan along with minced garlic
3.	Season with basil, pepper, oregano and salt. Cook for 5 minutes or until chicken start to turn golden
4.	Spiralize zucchini while chicken is cooking. You can use a spiralizer or simply use a vegetable peeler to make ribbons of zucchini
5.	Add crushed tomato and leave to simmer for about 5 minutes.
6.	Roast cashews in an oven or in a pan until it turns golden. Season with salt, turmeric and paprika
7.	Add spiralized zoodles and cherry tomatoes then add more salt to season if needed. Cook for 1 more minutes then remove from meat
8.	Serve chicken zoodles with the spiced cashews & fresh basil

Time: 25 Minutes | Amount: 4 to 6 servings
Calories: 487.7kcal | Carbs: 7.3g | Protein:34g | Fat: 36g

Ingredients

- Olive oil (2 tablespoons)
- Chicken breasts (boneless)-thinly sliced (1.5lbs/0/7kg)
- Heavy cream (1c)
- Chicken broth (1/2c)
- Italian seasoning and Garlic powder (1 teaspoon each)
- Parmesan cheese (1/2c)
- Chopped spinach (1 c)
- Dried tomatoes (1/2c)

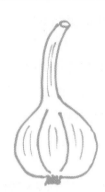

How to prepare

1.	Cook chicken in oil in a large skillet over medium to high heat for 3-5 minutes on both sides until it turns golden brown with no pink in its center.
2.	Once done, remove the chicken then set aside.
3.	Whisk heavy cream, garlic powder, chicken broth, parmesan and italian seasoning together over medium to high heat until it begins to thicken.
4.	Add spinach and the sun-dried tomatoes. Leave to simmer until spinach begins to wilt. Return chicken to pan then serve. May be served with pasta if desired

Time: 20 minutes | Amount: 4 servings

Calories: 230 kcal | Carbs:11g | Protein: 30g | Fat: 9g

Ingredients

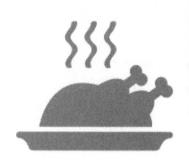

- Turkey Tenderloin (1 lb/0.45kg)- cut into steaks (1/4 inch thick)
- Salt (1 teaspoon)-divided
- Olive oil(2 tablespoons)divided
- Sweet onion (1/2, large) sliced
- Yellow and red bell pepper (1 each)- cut into strips
- Ground fresh black pepper (1/4 tsp)
- Italian seasoning (1/2 tsp)
- Red wine vinegar (2 tsp)
- Tomatoes crushed (1, 14 oz/396g)-fire roasted

For Garnish

- Fresh chopped parsley or basil (optional)

How to prepare

1.	Sprinkle salt over turkey (1/2 teaspoon).
2.	Heat oil (1 tbsp) in a large skillet over medium to high heat. Cook half of the turkey in this for about 1-3 minutes or till lightly browned. Flip turkey& continue cooking until cooked through.
3.	Remove turkey and transfer to a plate. Cover with a foil to keep warm. Repeat the same process for the remaining turkey.
4.	Add onions, bell peppers, & 1/2 teaspoon of oil to skillet, cover & cook for about 5-7 minutes. Until onions & peppers are softened. Remove the lid & stir once in a while as you cook.
5.	Increase heat to medium to high, add some Italian seasoning and the peppers. Continue to cook until for about 30 seconds and stir regularly. Add the red wine vinegar and cook for about 20 seconds until it is almost evaporated completely. Add in the tomatoes and leave to simmer for a while.
6.	Add the turkey to the skillet. Also, pour in any of the juice that are accumulated on the plate. Reduce heat to medium to low and leave to cook for about 2 minutes turning occasionally in the sauce.
7.	Serve with toppings.

LOW CARB TURKEY AND PEPPERS

Time: 30 minutes | Amount: 4 servings
Calories: 293 kcal | Carbs :6g | Proteins:25g | Fat: 17g

Ingredients

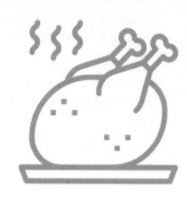

- Chicken breast (1.5 lbs/0.75g)
- Garam masala (2 tablespoon)
- Fresh grated ginger (2 tablespoons)
- Plain yogurt (4 oz)
- Minced garlic (3 teaspoons)
- Coconut oil (1 tablespoon)
- For the Sauce:
- Butter or ghee (2 tablespoons)
- Fresh ginger (2 teaspoons) grated
- 1 onion
- Ground coriander (1 tablespoon)
- Crushed tomatoes (14.5 oz/411g)
- Cumin (2 teaspoons)
- Heavy cream (1/2 cup)
- Garam masala (1/2 tablespoon)
- Salt (added to taste)
- Cilantro and cauliflower rice (Optional)

How to prepare

1.	Cut chicken to smaller pieces (2 inches per piece) & place in a bowl. Add 2 tablespoon of garam masala, grated ginger, minced garlic and yogurt. Stir to mix and leave to chill for 30 minutes.
2.	Blend the Ingredients for the sauce in a blender until smooth and set aside.
3.	In a skillet over medium heat, add 1 tbsp of oil then place chicken and marinade. Cook for about 3 to 4 minutes on each side till it is browned. Add the sauce then cook for 6 more minutes
4.	Stir in ghee & heavy cream then cook for 1 additional minute.
5.	Can be topped with cilantro and served with cauliflower rice.

Time: 35 Minutes | Amount: 4 servings

Calories:142kcal | Carbs: 4g | Protein: 7g | Fat: 11g

Ingredients

- Cauliflower rice (3 cups)
- 1 egg (beaten)
- Almond meal (1/2c)
- Diced onion (1/2c)
- Parmesan (1/2 cup + more for topping)
- Mozzarella cheese (1/4c)
- Garlic powder (1/2 teaspoon)
- Chopped chives (2 tablespoon)
- Pepper and salt (added to taste)

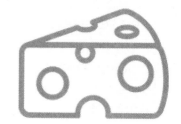

How to prepare

1.	Preheat oven to about 375oF/180oC
2.	Mix cauliflower rice, onion, almond, egg, mozzarella, Parmesan, garlic powder and chives then add salt and ground pepper to season and stir.
3.	Form tots from the mixture. Place them on prepared baking sheet with an even space between them.
4.	Sprinkle extra Parmesan cheese on each tot (optional)
5.	Bake in preheated oven for 20 minutes till it turns a golden brown color. Check about halfway through baking.

Time:20 minutes | Amount: 4 servings

Calories: 742 kcal | Carbs:6g | Proteins: 42g | Fats: 60g

Ingredients

- 2 eggs
- Pouring cream (1 tablespoon)
- Parmesan cheese (1/2 cup) finely grated
- Almond meal (1 1/2 cups)
- Continental parsley (1/3 cup) finely chopped
- Chilli flakes (optional) 1 teaspoon
- 2 avocados
- 2 zucchini (large, cut into wedges)
- Rice bran oil (1/3 cup)
- Salad leaves and lemon wedges (to serve)

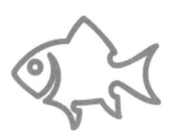

How to prepare

1.	Preheat oven to 400oF/200oC. Prepare baking tray by lining with a large baking paper
2.	Whisk eggs & cream in a bowl. Add 1 tablespoon to this. In another shallow bowl mix almond meal, cheese, parsley, rind & chilli flakes.
3.	Halve avocado and remove stone, then peel skin away & cut into wedges (about 6 to 8).
4.	Coat each piece of avocado in egg mixture. Let the excess drip off then coat with the almond meal mixture. Repeat this with the zucchini and fish as well.
5.	Spread avocado and zucchini on the tray. Place fish on a plate. Cover it all up & place in fridge for about 10 minutes.
6.	Spray zucchini and avocado with some oil & place in oven. Leave to bake for 20 minutes or until it turns crisp and golden
7.	Cook fish in oil in a large frying pan over medium to high heat pan for 2 to 3 minutes.
8.	To be served with lemon wedges and salad leaves.

Time: 1 hour | Amount:8 servings

Calories:339kcal | Carbs: 4g | Protein: 24g | Fat: 24g

Ingredients

- Olive oil (1 tablespoon)
- Minced chicken (500g/17g)
- 1 leek (trimmed and thinly sliced)
- Punnet button mushrooms (200g/7oz) sliced
- English spinach (1 bunch) rinsed, trimmed, dried and chopped
- Cream cheese (250g/8oz packet)
- Dried tarragon (1 tsp)
- Tomato pasta sauce (1/2 c)
- Coarsely grated mozzarella
- Cauliflower lasagne sheets
- Trimmed cauliflower (coarsely chopped)
- Parmesan (Finely grated) 1/2 c
- 2 eggs

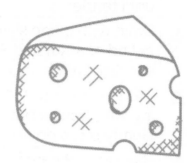

How to prepare

1.	For cauliflower lasagne sheets: process cauliflower in food processor. Transfer this to a microwave-safe bowl. Cover and warm up in a microwave oven for 8 minutes. Stir occasionally until tender.
2.	Drain with a fine sieve. Press down using a wooden spoon to get rid of any liquid. Return to bowl and add eggs and Parmesan. Stir well to mix.
3.	Preheat oven to 180oC/375oF. Prepare 2 baking trays by lining with baking paper. Divide the cauliflower into the 2 trays. Gently press down to form rectangles.
4.	Bake in preheated oven for 20 minutes or until mixture dries out. Remove, then set aside to cool. Cut into 6 lasagna sheets once cooled.
5.	Meanwhile, in a frying pan, heat oil and add leek then turn the heat down and leave it to cook for 4 minutes till it is soft.
6.	Turn heat back up. Add the chicken then cook for 10 additional minutes. Add mushroom at the five minutes mark and continue to cook. Add spinach and cook for 5 minutes until spinach wilts. Finally, add cream cheese & cook for about 2 minutes till cream melt.
7.	Grease baking dish and brush its base lightly with some tomato pasta sauce (use half). place 2 pieces of the lasagne over sauce. Top this with 1/2 of chicken mixture then sprinkle with mozzarella.
8.	Add another layer of cauliflower using the remaining chicken and the remaining lasagne, mozzarella and pasta sauce.
9.	Bake for about 30 minutes until it turns golden. Set this aside to cool (about 7 minutes) before serving.

Time: 25 minutes | Amount: 4 servings

Calories: 684kcal | Carbs:7g | Protein: 32g | Fat:57g

Ingredients

Macadamia oil (2 tablespoons)

Chicken thigh fillets (600g/1.3lbs) cut into small (3cm pieces)

Brown onion (1, sliced)

Garlic cloves (2, crushed)

Fresh ginger (2 teaspoons, finely grated)

Red chillies (2, finely chopped) extra for serving

Turmeric (1/2 teaspoon)

Brown Mustard seeds (2 teaspoons)

Ground cumin (2 teaspoon)

Ground coriander (1 teaspoon)

Coconut cream (400ml)

Broccoli (500g/1lb)

Lime juice and fish sauce (to taste)

Baby spinach leaves (100g/3.5oz)

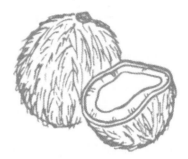

How to prepare

1.	Heat some oil over high heat in a saucepan.
2.	Add half of the chicken and cook for 2-3 until it is browned. Transfer to plate and repeat this for the remaining chicken.
3.	Add the rest of the oil and onions to the pan then cook for 3-4 minutes until softened. Add garlic, chilli, mustard seeds, coriander, turmeric, & cumin then cook for 2 minutes.
4.	Add coconut cream and chicken and bring to boil. Cover partially, turn down the heat and leave to simmer for 15-20 minutes or until chicken becomes tender.
5.	Process broccoli in a processor until it is finely chopped. Transfer broccoli to microwave-safe bowl. Heat in microwave for about 2 minutes to tenderize meat. Remove from heat and season with some lime juice & fish sauce. Sprinkle with spinach and extra chilli. To be served with broccoli rice.

Time: 20 minutes | Amount: 8 servings
Calories: 345kcal | Carbs:6g | Protein: 23g | Fat: 25g

Ingredients

Full fat Greek yogurt (1/4 cup)

Blue cheese crumbles (1/2 cup)

Juice (from 1/2 lemon)

Chicken breasts (2, cooked and shredded)

Romaine lettuce leaves (8, large and sturdy)

Walnuts (2 tablespoons) toasted & crumbled

Raspberries (8, split in half)

Chives (2 teaspoons) sliced into pieces of 1/4 inch each.

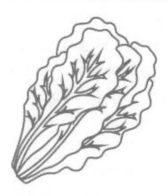

How to prepare

1.	Mix yogurt & blue cheese in a bowl then add the lemon juice as preferred.
2.	Add in the chicken pieces and stir until they are fully coated
3.	Add more yogurt, blue cheese & more lemon (if needed)
4.	Spoon the coated chicken shred onto the center of the romaine lettuce leaves. Divide meat equally between them. Place on a rimmed baking sheet or cutting board and set upright next to each other.
5.	Sprinkle walnut pieces, chives, and raspberry halves between lettuce leaves and serve immediately.

Time: 40 minutes | Amount: 2-3 servings

Calories: - | Carbs: - | Protein: - | Fat: -

Ingredients

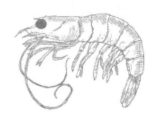

- 2 limes
- Red bell pepper (1 seeded & julienned)
- Large yellow onion (1/2, sliced thinly)
- Canola oil (2 teaspoons + 1/3 cup)
- Garlic cloves (2)
- Kosher salt (1 tsp)
- Chilli powder (1/2 tsp)
- Ground cumin (1/4 teaspoon)
- Oregano (1/2 tsp, dried)
- Raw shrimp (de-viened and shelled)-1 lb/0.45kg
- Cayenne pepper (1/2 tsp)
- 6 flour tortillas
- Mexican crema (or Greek yogurt)

How to prepare

1.	Preheat oven to about 400oF/202oC.
2.	Juice 1/2 of the lime and cut the other half into six wedges and set aside
3.	Toss onion and bell peppers into 2 teaspoons of canola oil to coat it. Scatter them onto a prepared sheet pan.
4.	Pour the lime juice into the blender, add the remaining oil, salt, and spices. Pulse the blender once to mix. Marinate shrimp in a large zip lock bag for about 15 minutes. Toss occassionally to coat.
5.	Roast bell peppers and onion for about 10 minutes
6.	Remove shrimp from marinade and polka dot onto sheet pan of roasted veggies. Roast this for about 8 minutes or more until it turns pink and fragrant.
7.	Heat flour tortillas and set out mexican creama along with the lime wedges to serve

SHEET PAN SHRIMP FAJITAS RECIPE

Time: 45 minutes | Amount: 6-8 servings

Calories:311kcal | Carbs: 11g | Protein: 11g | Fat:13g

Ingredients

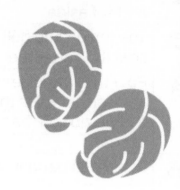

- Extra-virgin olive oil (3 to 4 teaspoons)
- Brussels spouts (2 lbs) halved
- Kosher salt (1/2 teaspoon)
- Bacon (4 to 6 ounces) cut into 1/4 inch size
- Onion (1 cup, diced)
- Heavy cream (about 2 cups)
- Sour cream (1/2 cup)
- Smoked gouda cheese (8 oz/226g, grated)
- Feta cheese (for garnish) 4oz/113g
- Low moisture mozzarella cheese (8 oz/226g, grated)
- Garlic salt (1 teaspoon)
- Black pepper

How to prepare

1.	Heat 3 to 4 teaspoons of olive oil in a shallow skillet over medium heat
2.	Carefully place Brussels sprouts in the pan once the oil is hot. Do not stir at first. Cook like this for about 15 minutes. Stir once in a while to ensure that the sprouts are charred on most of its sides. Once done, remove and set this aside.
3.	To the pan, add bacon and saute for 5 minutes. Stir constantly until the bacon become slightly crispy.
4.	Remove the bacon and set aside in a plate.
5.	Reduce heat. Add onion to bacon fat in the skillet and saute for 5 additional minute. Stir regularly until the onions become softened and slightly caramelized.
6.	Add in the sour cream, heavy cream, mozzarella, gouda and feta cheese then stir to mix. Turn the heat down to low once the cheese melts.
7.	Return the brussels sprouts back to skillet with the cheese sauce. Stir till it is well combined. You can add in more heavy cream if the sauce is too thick. Add the garlic salt & pepper to season.
8.	Serve garnished with reserved bacon and serve immediately.

3-CHEESE BRUSSELS SPROUTS RECIPE

Time:1 hour | Amount: 4 yields

Calories: 563kcal | Carbs:35g | Protein: 42g | Fat:31g

Ingredients

♦ Mixed greens (2 cups)
♦ Diced tomato (1, large)
♦ Chopped fresh parsley (1/4c)
♦ Kalamata olives (10, large) all pitted
♦ Zucchini (1, small) sliced lengthwise
♦ Diced avocado (1/2)
♦ Green onion (1 sliced)
♦ Light tuna (1 can) drained
♦ Extra-virgin olive oil (1 tablespoon)
♦ Balsamic vinegar (1 tablespoon)
♦ Fine sea salt (1/4 tsp)
♦ Black pepper (1/4 teaspoon)

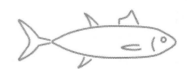

How to prepare

1.	Grill the zucchini slices in a sizzling hot skillet grill pan. Grill on both sides.
2.	Remove from pan. Leave for some minutes to cool.
3.	Cut into smaller pieces.
4.	Combine all the ingredient in a mixing bowl. Stir delicately until it is all well combined
5.	Serve immediately

Time: 45 minutes | Amount: 2 servings

Calories: 661 kcal | Carbs:4g | Protein: 27g | Fat:59g

Ingredients

- Cauliflower (1/2 head, medium)
- Eggs (2, large)
- Garlic cloves (2, chopped)
- Pork belly (100g/3.5 oz)
- green capsicums (2, mini)
- Spring onions (2)
- Tamari (1 tbsp)/ soy sauce
- Picked ginger (1 tsp)
- Black sesame seeds (1 teaspoon)

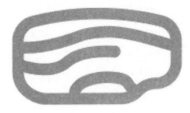

How to prepare

1.	Chop cauliflower into florets. Place florets in the food processor then Pulse till rice-sized granules are formed. (don't overdo it to avoid ending up with mashed cauliflower)
2.	Heat oil for some seconds in a frying pan. Add cauliflower then saute for about 5 minutes. Once cooked, remove from pan & set aside.
3.	Prepare omelette by beating eggs and adding to the frying pan. Swirl around to thin out the omelette.Flip, & cook for 1 additional minute once cooked though. Remove from the pan. Set this aside also.
4.	To the frying pan, add garlic and cooked for some seconds until fragrant
5.	Add in the pork belly, slice omelette into small cubes while this is cooking.
6.	Add capsicum and half of the spring onion to the pork belly once it is cooked through. Cook for 1 additional minute
7.	Return cauliflower and diced egg back into the pan. Add soy sauce & stir to mix.
8.	Cook until well combined over high heat.
9.	To be served steaming hot garnished with spring onion, picked ginger and sesame seeds.

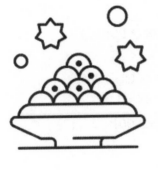

Time: 1 hour | Amount: 20 servings
Calories: 116kcal | Carbs: 7g | Protein:3g | Fat:10g

Ingredients

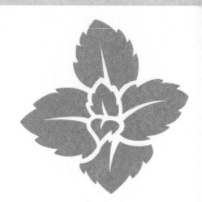

For cookies

♦ Almond flour (1 3/4c)

♦ Swerve sweetener (1/3c)

♦ Salt (1/4 tsp)

♦ Cocoa powder (1/3c)

♦ Vanilla extract (1/2 tsp)

♦ 1 large egg

♦ Baking powder (1 tsp)

For coating

♦ Coconut oil, or cocoa butter or butter (1 tbsp)

♦ Sugar-free dark chocolate or Lily's dark chocolate (200g/7 oz) chopped

♦ Peppermint extract (1 teaspoon)

How to prepare

1.	Preheat oven to 300oF/150oC. Prepare 2 baking sheets by lining with parchment papers
2.	Mix almond flour, sweetener, cocoa powder,salt, and baking powder in a bowl. Add in eggs, vanilla extract, and butter & mix well till dough is well mixed
3.	Roll out the dough between the 2 pieces of parchment paper to your desired thickness. Life off the top piece of the parchment paper then set aside
4.	Using a cookie cutter (2-inch diameter) cut out dough into circles and lift off gently. Place cookies on baking sheet. (you can gather up any leftover scraps and roll again)
5.	Bake cookies in the oven until it is firm to touch (20 to 30 minutes). Remove from oven then set aside to cool.
6.	To prepare chocolate coating, place a metal bowl over a pot of water simmering on medium to high heat. The bowl should not touch the water.
7.	Melt oil and chocolate in the bowl, stir till smooth & remove from heat. Stir in peppermint extract.
8.	Dip cookies into this chocolate mixture. Turn over using 2 forks until the cookie is fully coated. Remove, then place on a prepared baking sheet.
9.	Refrigerate until fully set.

Time: 1 hour | Amount: 24 servings

Calories: 375 kcal | Carbs: 17g | Protein: 14.5g | Fat: 29.5g

Ingredients

- ◆ Almond flour (1 1/3 c)
- ◆ Fine sea salt (1/4 teaspoon)
- ◆ Ghee or grass-fed butter (1/3c + 1 teaspoon)
- ◆ Coconut flour (1 tbsp)
- ◆ Erythritol monk fruit blend (4 tablespoons)
- ◆ Vanilla extract (1/2 teaspoon)
- ◆ Collagen peptides (1 tablespoon)
- ◆ Vanilla shortbread protein bar (1, crumbled)

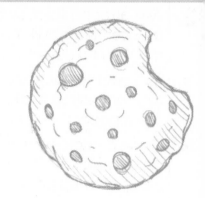

How to prepare

1.	Mix all the ingredient for the shortbread except the collagen bar in a food processor
2.	Remove dough and spread using a rolling pin until thickness is about 3.5 mm
3.	Cut out the cookies using a round cutter, then refrigerate for about 30 minutes
4.	Preheat oven to about 170oC/350oF. Prepare perforated baking tray by lining it with silicone liner or parchment paper.
5.	Place frozen cookies on this baking sheet. Bake for 8 minutes or till it begins to turn golden. (time may vary based on thickness of the cookies, and the type of oven and baking tray used.
6.	Remove from oven, cool then add chocolate glaze and collagen bar crumbs.

Time: 35 Minutes | Amount:24 servings

Calories: 86 kcal | Carbs:2g | Protein: 1g | Fat: 8g

Ingredients

Almond flour (144 g/5oz)

Cocoa powder (37 g/1.5oz)

Kosher salt (3/4 teaspoon)

Black cocoa powder (13g/0.5oz) (you can also use regular cocoa)

Xanthan gum (1/2 teaspoon)

Baking soda (1/2 teaspoon)

Espresso powder (1/4 teaspoon) optional

Grass fed butter (80g/6oz) unsalted

Erythritol (128g/4Oz)

1 egg

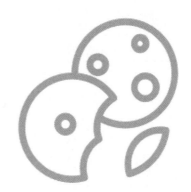

For the vanilla cream filling

Grass-fed butter (unsalted) 56g/2 oz

Coconut oil (14g)

Vanilla extract (1.5 teaspoon)

Kosher salt (a pinch)

Erythritol or any powdered sweetener (added to taste)

How to prepare

1.	Mix almond flour, xanthan gum, baking soda, cocoa powder espresso powder & salt in a bowl then set aside.
2.	Use an electric to cream butter in a large bowl for about 2 minutes. Add sweetener and mix some more till well mixed & the sweetener dissolves.
3.	Add egg & mix well until the mixture appears to be slightly broken (not thoroughly smooth)
4.	Add in half of flower mixture & mix on low until it is well mixed using a mixer. Add in the remaining portion of the mixture Wrap in cling film then refrigerate for 1 hour or overnight.
5.	Preheat oven to 350ºF/180ºC. Line baking tray with parchment paper
6.	Roll out the rough on 2 pieces of parchment paper. Spread out until it is thin, then cut out Oreos to a diameter of about 1 3/4 inches.
7.	Transfer cookies to the baking tray and refrigerate for about 15 minutes before you start baking. Bake in oven for about 12 minutes..
8.	Leave to cool for 10 minutes before transferring to cooling rack.
9.	Prepare vanilla cream filling, mix coconut oil and cream butter in a medium bowl using an electric mixer. To this, add vanilla extract,& a pinch of salt then mix well. Add the powdered sweetener to taste and mix thoroughly until the texture become fluffy.
10.	Spread cream onto a cookie and sandwich between another one. Refrigerate cookies until set.

Time: 5 Minutes | Amount: 8 servings

Calories: 329kcal | Carbs: 4g | Protein:2g | Fat: 29.6g

Ingredients

- Shredded coconut (unsweetened) 3 cups
- Coconut oil (3/8 cup)
- Xylitol (1/2 cup) or any other sweetner
- Vanilla (2 teaspoon)
- Salt (add as desired)

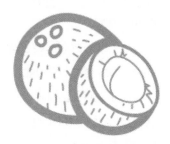

How to prepare

1.	Mix all Ingredients in a food processor or blender till they all stick together. (do nut turn your blender to high speed especially if it is high-powered)
2.	Remove mixture from food processor and form into any shape you desire then decorate with some shredded coconut, carob powder and/or cocoa, or crushed nuts. (you can leave plain too)
3.	Leave aside on a plate to firm up

Time: 26 minutes | Amount: 12 servings

Calories: 138 kcal | Carbs:4.6g | Protein: 4.4g | Fat: 11.4g

Ingredients

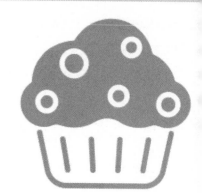

- Melted butter (110g/4oz)
- Granulated sweetener (any of your choice (4 tablespoon)
- Coconut flower (50g/2oz)
- Baking powder (1 teaspoon)
- Lemon juice (2 tablespoon)
- Lemon zest (2 tablespoon)
- Vanilla (1 teaspoon)
- Eggs (8, medium)
- Fresh blueberries (120g/5oz)

How to prepare

1.	Mix melted butter, coconut flower, sweetener, baking powder, lemon juice, vanilla and lemon zest
2.	Add eggs to this mixture. Do this one at a time and mixing in between each addition
3.	Taste batter to ensure sweetener and flavor is as desired and the subtle tast of coconut flour is masked.
4.	Divide mixture into the cupcake cups (12)
5.	Press in blueberries into each batter of cupcake.
6.	Bake in oven for about 15 minutes at 350oF/180oC until it turns begins to turn golden
7.	Cover with ream cheese frosting (lemon or vanilla flavor. Serve garnished with lemon zest and fresh blueberries.

Time: 5 minutes | Amount: 18 servings

Calories: 96 kcal | Carbs : 1.4g | Proteins: 1g | Fat: 12g

Ingredients

Coconut butter (1/2 cup)

Coconut oil (1/2 cup)

Cocoa powder (1/2 cup)

Any sweetener of choice

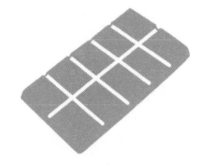

How to prepare

1.	Line a mini muffin tin with muffin liners then set aside
2.	Melt coconut oil over a stove or in a microwave. Add cocoa powder to the bowl of coconut oil and mix thoroughly until it is fully combined with no clumps remaining. You can add a sweetener if desired
3.	Coat the sides and bottom of the muffin liners with some melted chocolate. Keep some of the chocolate for later for topping.
4.	Place the muffin tins in the freezer for some minutes to firm up
5.	Divide butter into the cups and top with the remaining chocolate then freeze to firm.

Time: 45 Minutes | Amount: 12 servings

Calories: 208 kcal | Carbs: 8g | Protein: 4g | Fat: 18g

Ingredients

- Coconut oil (1/2c) melted
- Cold brewed coffee (1/2c)
- Cacao powder (3 tablespoons)
- Almond flour (1/2c)
- Cinnamon (1/2tsp)
- Baking soda (1tsp)
- Monk fruit extract (1/4 cup)- liquid
- Vanilla extract (1 teaspoon)
- Buttermilk (1.5 tbsp apple cider vinegar+ 0.5 cup almond milk)
- 2 eggs

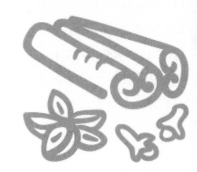

For Chocolate Avocado Frosting

- Avocado (1/2 large)
- Cacao powder (2 tablespoon)
- Coconut oil (1 tablespoon)
- Unsweetened coconut milk (1/4 cup)
- Monk fruit extract (2 teaspoons)

How to prepare

1.	Preheat oven to 400°F/202°C
2.	Mix coconut oil, cacao powder, cinnamon and cold brew in a mixing bowl
3.	Mix almond flour, baking soda, & monk fruit extract in a mixing bowl.
4.	Add buttermilk, eggs, & vanilla extract to the bowl of coconut oil then add this to almond flour
5.	Mix all until well combined either by hand or using an electric mixer.
6.	Bake batter for 20 minutes in a prepared baking sheet
7.	Remove from the oven and leave to cool while preparing frosting;
8.	Mix all the frosting Ingredients using a mixer until completely combined and smooth. A food processor or blender can be used for this.
9.	Spread frosting on the cake once it is cooled then cut it into slices and serve.

Time: 30 minutes | Amount: 6 Yields

Calories: 33 kcal | Carbs:2g | Proteins: 1g | Fats: 3g

Ingredients

- Avocados (2 , medium)
- Lemon juice (2 tablespoon)
- Sweetener-any sugar alternative (6 tablespoon)
- Almond milk (1 cup) unsweetened
- Chocolate ganache
- Cacao butter (2 teaspoon)
- Low carb chocolate (2/3 cup)

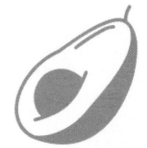

How to prepare

1.	In a mixer, place avocados, sugar alternative and lemon juice and combine thoroughly
2.	Fill all the Popsicle molds with this mixture and freeze
3.	Melt cacao butter and chocolate in a double container ther set aside to cool
4.	Dip each frozen Popsicle into cooled chocolate
5.	You can eat straightaway or return to the freezer for later.

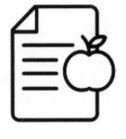

Time: 15 minutes | Amount: 3 servings

Calories: 244kcal | Carbs: 5g | Protein:5.5g | Fat:23g

Ingredients

- Coconut flour (1/2 c)
- Coconut oil (2 tbsp)
- Baking soda (1/2 tsp)
- 4 Pasture-raised eggs
- Vanilla (1 teaspoon)
- Ceylon cinnamon (1/2 tsp)
- Coconut cream (1/2 cup)
- Himalayan salt (1/4 tsp)
- Unsweetened almond milk (1/2c)
- Coconut oil or grass-fed ghee for cooking

How to prepare

1.	Add all Ingredients into a high-powered blender except the ghee. Turn on blender to mix until Ingredients are smoothly mixed. Scrape the sides of your blender if needed.
2.	Coat a medium sized skillet with ghee and place over medium heat. Pour about 1/2 cup of batter into heated skillet. Cook until one side turns golden then flip & continue cooking until the other side turns golden as well.
3.	Can be served immediately with berries, grass-fed ghee or any other keto-friendly topping or kept for later.

Time: 55 minutes | Amount: 12 servings

Calories: 345 kcal | Carbs: 5.5g | Protein: 11.2g | Fat: 30.5g

Ingredients

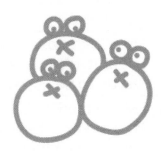

- Blanched almonds (1 cup)
- Flakedalmonds (1/4 cup)
- Brazil nuts (1/2 cup)
- Pecans(1/2 cup)
- Pumpkin seeds (1/2 cup)
- Sunflower seeds (1/2 cup)
- Chia seeds (3 tablespoons)
- Shelled hemp seeds (3 tbsp)
- Flax seeds (3 tablespoon)
- Unsweetened flaked coconut (1 cup)
- Blueberries (8.8oz/250g)
- Virgin coconut oil (1/4 cup)
- Vanilla bean powder (1 teaspoon)
- Whey protein powder (1/4 cup)
- Egg white (from 1 large egg)
- Sea salt (1/8 cup)
- Swerve or Erythritol (1/4 cup)

How to prepare

1.	Heat oven to about 300ºF/150 ºC. Chop almonds, brazil nuts and pecan & mix in a bowl. Also add the pumpkin seeds, chia, hemp seeds, and sunflower flax and mix.
2.	To this mixture, add the protein powder, vanilla, salt and erythritol.
3.	In a high speed blender, Blitz about 3/4 of your blueberries until it looks like a coulis. Keep the remaining blueberries aside to be used as topping,
4.	Mix blitzed blueberries with coconut oil and egg white. Spread the mix on a baking tray(12 x 8 inch/30 x 20 cm tray). add the remaining blueberries as toppings.
5.	Bake in oven for about 30 minutes. Add flaked coconut then bake for 8 more minutes until it turns golden.
6.	Remove the oven and leave to cool. Break it up with a fork and let it cool further.
7.	Can be served with yogurt, unsweetened almond milk, coconut whipped or sour cream. Can be stored refrigerated for about 5 days in a glass jar.

Time: 15 Minutes | Amount: 1 sandwich
Calories: 603 kcal | Carbs:7g | Protein: 22g | Fat: 54g

Ingredients

Sausage patties (2)

Egg (1 large)

Cream cheese (1 tablespoon)

Sharp cheddar (2 tablespoon)

Avocado (1/4 medium)

Sriracha (added to taste)

Salt & pepper (added to taste)

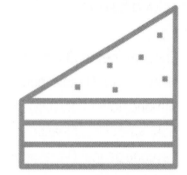

How to prepare

1.	Cook sausages skillet based on instructions on its package then set aside
2.	Place cream cheese & sharp cheddar in a bowl & microwave until it has melted.
3.	Mix srircha and cheese then set aside
4.	Mix eggs with the seasonings then make a small omelet.
5.	Fill omelette with the sriracha mixture and assemble into sandwich.
6.	Serve immediately or wrap sandwich in a plastic wrap and aluminum foil and refrigerate.

Time: 20 Minutes | Amount: 4 servings

Calories: 522kcal | Carbs: 6g | Protein:30g | Fat: 41g

Ingredients

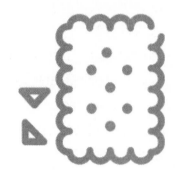

For cloud biscuit

♦ Egg (1)

♦ Cheddar cheese (3/4 cup)

♦ Heavy cream (1 tablespoon)

♦ Almond flour (4 oz/112g)

♦ Baking powder (1 teaspoon)

♦ Cayenne pepper (1 teaspoon

For toppings

♦ Smoked salmon (8 oz/ 250g)

♦ Red onion (2 tablespoon)

♦ Fresh dill (optional)

♦ Lemon juice

♦ Arugula (rocket)

How to prepare

1.	Heat oven to about 360oF/180°C
2.	Mix flour & cheese in a bowl. Add baking powder & cayenne pepper then stir
3.	Crack egg into another bowl & whisk.
4.	Make a hole at the center of the flour & cheese mixture then pour in the egg. Add cream an mix all together.
5.	Scoop mixture onto prepared baking sheet and form into patties
6.	Place patties in oven & bake for about 15 minutes. Remove from oven then leave to cool for about 2 minutes. Slice each biscuit into half
7.	To build sandwich , add cream cheese, salmon and other toppings. Assemble when it's time to eat.

Time: 26 minutes | Amount: 4 servings

Calories: 150 kcal | Carbs:2g | Protein: 3g | Fat: 14g

Ingredients

- Coconut oil (2 tablespoon)
- Peanut butter (3 oz/84g)
- Vanilla extract
- Cocoa powder (2 1/2 tsp)
- Almond flour (4 oz/112g)
- Chia seeds(2 1/2 teaspoon)
- Stevia (1/2 teaspoon)
- Coconut flakes (1 3/4 tablespoon)

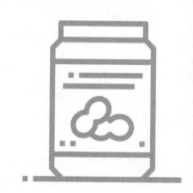

How to prepare

1.	Add peanut butter, cacao, vanilla extract, coconut oil and stevia in a bowl and mix
2.	Add chia seeds & almond flour then mix all thoroughly. Heat this mixture slightly for about 15 seconds if the mix is coming out dry and add a little coconut oil
3.	Spread the mixture on a baking sheet & place in a tray
4.	Freeze for about 20 minutes until it is solid
5.	Cut into chunks and dip in shredded coconut until a white coating is formed
6.	Store in a fridge till you are set to eat.

Time: 30 minutes | Amount: 4 servings

Calories: 610 kcal | Carbs :6 | Proteins:30g | Fat: 50g

ngredients

Chicken thigh (with bone and skin) 1 lb/0.45 kg

Sesame seeds (3 tablespoon)

Almond flour (4 oz/112g)

Red pepper flakes (not compulsory)

2 eggs

Broccoli (7 oz/ 220g)

Sea salt and pepper (added to taste)

Heavy cream (3 oz/84g)

For Garnish: red peppers (2 oz/54g),
sesame oil (about 2 tablespoon),
green onion (3 tablespoon),
soy sauce (3 tablespoon),
lime juice

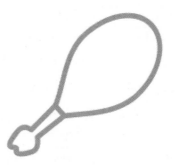

How to prepare

1.	Preheat oven. Add sesame seeds, sea salt, pepper and almond flour into a bowl mix well then add some chilli flakes (if desired)
2.	In another bowl, crack egg and add heavy cream then whisk
3.	Dip the chicken thighs first into the egg mixture then in the sesame mix. Do this for all the chicken thighs.
4.	Cook in oven for about 30 minutes
5.	Steam or boil broccoli for about 4 minutes until firm. Remove & place them in cold water.
6.	Remove the chicken thighs from oven and drizzle soil soy sauce and sesame oil over it.
7.	Serve chicken with the steamed veggies and sprinkle with sliced spring onions or any other topping of choice
8.	Cool, cover and refrigerate to store.

Time: 45 Minutes | Amount: 4servings

Calories: 571 kcal | Carbs:7g | Protein: 34g | Fat: 45g

ngredients

strip steak (12 oz/ 340g)0- cut into strips

Mushrooms & onions (3 oz/ 84g each)

Oregano (1 teaspoon)

Olive oil (3 tbsp)

Provolone cheese or cheddar (5 oz/140g)

Bell pepper (5 oz/140g)

Jalapeno (1 oz/28g)

Cream cheese (4 oz/112g)

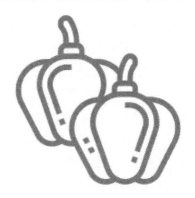

or Salad

Olive oil (2 tablespoon)

Lettuce (6 oz/170g)

Cherry tomatoes (3 oz/84g)

How to prepare

1.	Preheat oven to 400oF/202oC
2.	Chop the top of the bell pepper to remove its insides
3.	On a baking tray, place bell peppers then spray with some olive oil. Place in the oven & bake for 20 minutes.
4.	Place pan on medium to high heat, add onion and olive oil and fry until they become translucent
5.	Add more oil, then add steak, oregano and mushrooms. Cook till steak is done
6.	Add the steak and mushroom mix and cream cheese to the cooked bell pepper. Add more jalapeno, steak and provolone or cheddar cheese to top
7.	Do this for all the bell peppers. Return to oven and boil or grill for 5 minutes till cheese melts
8.	Cut into small portions and arrange in a meal prep containers along with lettuce and cherry tomato salad. Leave to cool before covering and storing containers in your refrigerator.

Time:50 minutes | Amount: 4 Yields

Calories: 378 kcal | Carbs:6g | Proteins: 32g | Fats: 21g

ingredients

or Chicken

- Chicken breast (with bone and skin removed) (1 lb/0.45kg)
- Pepper and salt (added to taste)
- Olive oil (2 tablespoon)
- Lime juice (1/4 cup)
- Freshly chopped cilantro (1/3 cup)
- Sea salt (1/8 teaspoon)
- Minced garlic (2 teaspoons)
- Honey (1/2 teaspoon)

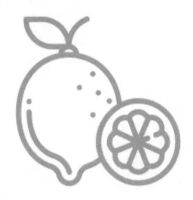

or Cauliflower Rice

- Olive oil (2 tablespoons)
- Cauliflower rice (3 cups)
- Ground cumin (1 teaspoon)
- Sea salt (1/8 cup)
- Garlic powder (2 teaspoons)
- Black beans (1/2 cup)
- Red onions (1/4 cup)
- Cherry tomatoes (1 cup)-halved

How to prepare

1.	Heat olive oil in a large skillet over medium heat.
2.	To this, add chicken & cook for 5-8 minutes on each side
3.	Leave to cool for 15-20 minutes before you slice and set aside
4.	Add the remaining Ingredients for the chicken into a bowl then mix
5.	Place chicken in this bowl & toss until it is well coated then refrigerate
6.	To prepare cauliflower rice, heat olive oil in a skillet then add the riced cauliflower and the spices then cook for about 5 minutes. Add black beans then saute for 2 additional minutes. Add in red onions then mix.
7.	Place chicken, cauliflower rice & tomatoes in a bowl & enjoy.

Time: 22 Minutes | Amount: 4 meals
Calories: 248kcal | Carbs:3.5g | Protein: 16g | Fat: 19g

ngredients

Bacon (8 slices)

Asparagus (8 large spears)

Greens (probably arugula) (4 cups)

Hard boiled eggs (4, large)

Berries (optional)

Lemon wedges (optional)

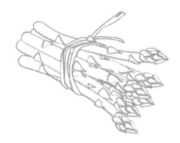

ow to prepare

1.	Preheat oven to 370oF/180oC
2.	Take each of asparagus spear and warp with a slice of bacon. You may bunch 2 or 3 together is spears are too small and wrap
3.	Add the bacon wrapped asparagus to a baking tray then broil for about 7 minutes. Flip and cook for about 3 to 7 more minutes or till bacon is done to your preference
4.	Remove from oven & add to a salad along with hard boiled egg & berries. Cna also be served with lemon wedge or stored for later.

Time: 35 minutes | Amount: 4 servings

Calories: 632 kcal | Carbs:15g | Protein: 49g | Fat: 43g

Ingredients

- Ground beef-pastured (3/4 lbs/0.3kg)
- Minced garlic (2 cloves)
- Yellow onion (1, divided)
- Dried thyme (1 teaspoon)
- Pepper and salt (added to taste)
- Dried oregano (1 teaspoon)
- chilli flakes (1/2 teaspoon-optional)
- grass-fed ghee or coconut oil (2 tablespoons)
- 1 avocado- sliced
- Arugula
- Top-quality pastured bacon (4 slices)

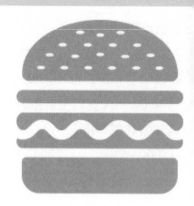

How to prepare

1.	Divide the yellow onions into quarters, dice one of the quarters then cut the rest into slices and set aside.
2.	Combine chopped onions with ground beef, garlic and the spices in a bowl. Mix well. Divide this mixture into 4 parts and form each one into patties
3.	add oil or ghee into a frying pan and swirl until the pan is well coated
4.	Heat pan then add patties. Cook both sides until browned
5.	While burgers are cooking, add remaining onions to the pan. Salt the slices and stir occasionally until caramelized.
6.	Add bacon slices into the same or different pans and cook till slightly crisp
7.	Divide the arugula between two plates, top with patties, onions and avocado slices
8.	Serve warm or store for later.

KETO HAMBURGER SALAD

EXCLUSIVE BONUS!

Get Keto Audiobook for FREE NOW!*

*The Ultimate Keto Diet Guide 2019-2020:
How to Loose weight with Quick and Easy Steps*

SCAN ME

or go to

www.free-keto.co.uk

*Listen free for 30 Days on Audible (for new members only)

The opinions and ideas of the author contained in this publication are designed to educate the reader in an informative and helpful manner. While we accept that the instructions will not suit every reader, it is only to be expected that the recipes might not gel with everyone. Use the book responsibly and at your own risk. This work with all its contents, does not guarantee correctness, completion, quality or correctness of the provided information. Always check with your medical practitioner should you be unsure whether to follow a low carb eating plan. Misinformation or misprints cannot be completely eliminated. Human error is real!

Picture: YARUNIV Studio // www.shutterstock.com

Design: Natalia Design